CONTENTS

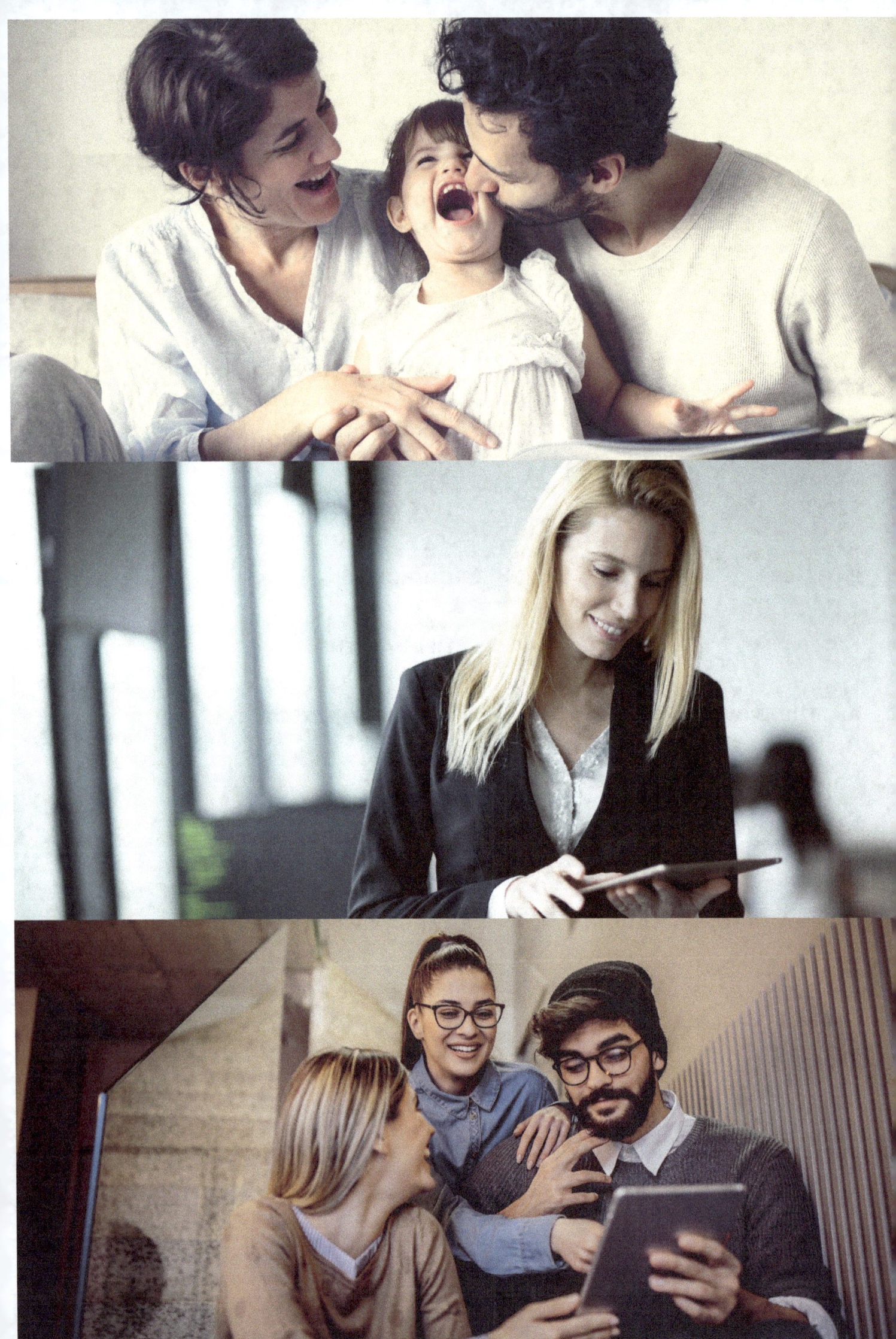

INTRODUCTION

According to the American College of Gastroenterology, 10-15% of all Americans suffer from IBS. Statistics indicate that it is the most common disorder diagnosed by gastroenterologists and primary care doctors.

Individuals living with chronic digestive disorders often wish they could be free of the demands of these conditions.

And they often find that doctors offer medication intended to mask symptoms rather than treat the root cause of their condition. While the last year has shown us how much we owe the nation's doctors, there are still many patients who -- rightly - complain that their medical consultations seem rushed, and they report that preventive measures are rarely discussed.

Samantha Wyland is one of those patients.

After a 20-year career as a ballet dancer, and following a miscarriage at the age of 34, Samantha's digestive issues took a turn for the worst, throwing her into early menopause and rendering her non-functional for two years. In the midst of her second part-time career in sales, this experience served as a wake-up call that the medical establishment did not have all the answers she needed to live a full and satisfying life.

Determined to control her health and support her family, she researched and educated her doctors about the root cause of her condition so that they may serve other patients more effectively. In 2019, Samantha enrolled in the Institute for Integrative Nutrition and became certified in this field. During her self-study and coursework, Samantha learned approaches for handling stress and poor diet, as well as a greater understanding of the importance of exercise and physical activity.

Making appropriate diet and lifestyle changes, managing stress, and noting common triggers will make traveling and spending quality time with family and friends more enjoyable without the fear and shame around digestive disorders such as diarrhea, constipation, gas, bloating and pain.

Armed with this knowledge, Samantha has had an opportunity to educate her doctors about the root cause of her condition so they may serve other patients more effectively.

Having found numerous life-changing insights and information that she has used to achieve the quality of life she dreamed of, Samantha is now dedicated to helping people whose careers, family time and social interactions are limited due to their fear and shame around their chronic digestive disorders.

AUTHOR'S NOTE

I want to share my real-life girl-next door journey of overcoming a functional digestive disorder (IBS). And that means rather than just rehashing some boring medical jargon, I want to tell you all the things I wish I knew 7 years ago that no one told me.

I hope you will take away some inspiration and practical information, something you would not have found elsewhere, and that these pages will be a new beginning for you. That you will look at your condition with fresh eyes filled with hope.

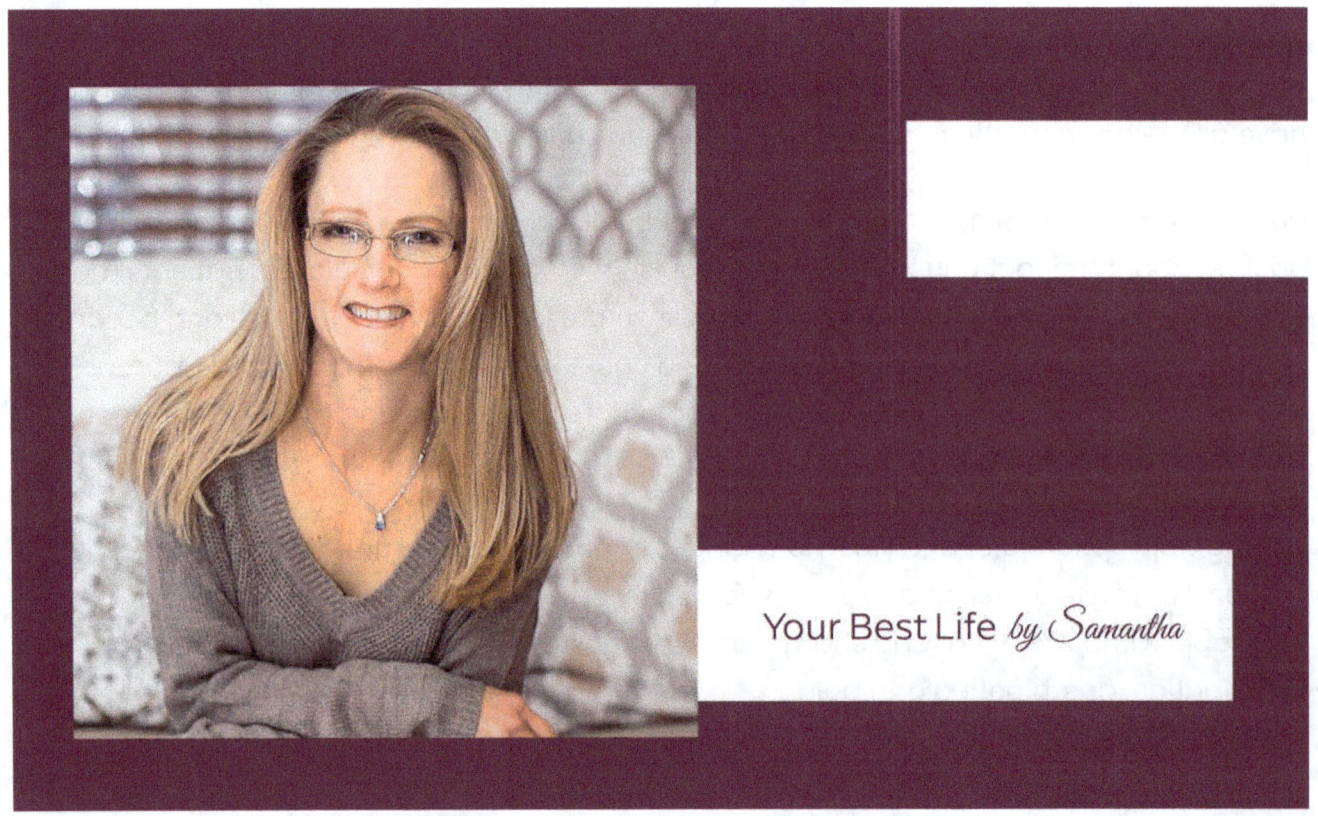

Your Best Life *by Samantha*

KNOCKED OUT

I was in a near-fatal accident in my late teens. I didn't see the white light or anything, but it was pretty bad. My lifelong dream at the time was to be a ballerina. I had been studying intensely for many years. After multiple skull fractures and a damaged inner ear, my doctors told me the accident was the end of that dream.

After multiple surgeries and the green light from my neurologist, I went back to taking classes. What did I have to lose? I remember standing at the ballet barre. I can only imagine what a hot mess I looked like. I had facial paralysis and stitches down the right side of my head. The teacher walked over to me, looked me in the eyes for a moment, kissed my forehead, and continued with class.

I don't remember how well I danced in those early days of my recovery. I didn't fall or crash into anyone that I am aware of. Maybe it was fantastic. Who knows?

I obtained a BA in Dance from a small university and had an incredible 20-year teaching career. I was no Misty Copeland, but I had a good run.

Looking back, I believe this was possible because I went right back to dancing. I didn't wait until I looked like myself again. I retrained my body to dance as I healed. The more I danced, the more I adjusted to my "new normal."

I used that same tenacity to get control of my IBS. If I could dance after a head trauma, I was confident I could stop my suffering.

Was there a time in your life when someone told you your dreams were impossible, and you did it anyway?

EXPERTS

I do not believe the title "MD" makes a doctor an expert on YOU. Specialists run tests, prescribe medications. Surgeons do surgery. They all have hundreds of patients. Not one of them is like you.

My facial paralysis is a perfect example of this. At one of the lowest points of my life, I found myself with two theories presented to me:

A. My facial plastic Dr - Wait and see if the swelling around the nerve goes down, allowing it to function again.

B. Hotshot Neurosurgeon - Have major brain surgery to repair the nerve that may or may not be cut.

"Umm - I'll take A for 100, Alex."

I believe in doctors, medicine, and surgery. I wouldn't be alive without them. If my face had not regained movement, I might have considered surgery. Just not with the jerk with a god complex that presented it as the only option.

Was the waiting scary? You bet. Making decisions about your own health takes a HUGE leap of faith.

Ex 2 - I was having major digestive issues in my late 30s. I was going around and around between my GP, Gastro, and OBGYN. I was at an OB appointment telling her about my pain and digestive issues.

"Yup - it's just gonna be that way at your age." Maybe she had PMS that day, but I was not about to accept that I would feel this way forever.

"Wait, hold my beer."

Back to my gastro with the same story. He had the answer I needed at the time.

Many, many appointments, many different options. Listen to your inner voice. Be an advocate for your own health!!

You do you!

"SAMANTHA, YOU HAVE A VERY NICE LIFE."

ENTITLED

I used to think I deserved certain exceptions - like the world owed me after all I went through.

If I did a favor for someone or supported them, I expected it in return.

This pissed off many people in my life, and I realized I was living with a victim mentality. Hearing the words come out of my mouth as I was screaming at a former colleague and friend, I realized what a spoiled brat I was.

He calmly replied to my tirade:

"Samantha, you have a very nice life."

That attitude had to go ASAP, and when I started to look at all the good things I had in my life and how I had busted my butt to get there, the victim mentality began to fade away.

The truth is no one owes you squat.

If you want to change something in your life or your health, you need to get off your behind and find a solution.

BUT you don't have to row the boat alone. There is a solution to every problem, and if you find the right people to support you, the solution will present itself.

FACEPALM

Anyone that knows me knows I am somewhat of a coffee snob. Dunkin, Starbucks, Lattes, oh my! It must be fresh. If it has been on the burner for more than 30 minutes, I will request a fresh pot. (Servers love me.)

To make matters worse, my husband worked for a distributor of single-cup coffee pods and brewers. All the sudden, we were getting FREE coffee for life.

I was a three cup a day girl for as long as I can remember. I also had panic attacks, bathroom issues, and trouble sleeping.

Coffee had to go. It felt like losing my best friend. All that free coffee was staring me in the face, mocking me. I dialed it back to 2 cups a day. Halfway through my second cup one morning, the heart palpitations, shaking and sweating began.

Dumped that cup right down the drain. In addition to other diet and lifestyle changes, I was able to keep my 1 cup of morning magic and swap out the rest for green tea.

Giving up something you love is dang hard but sometimes necessary for your health.

What habit do you KNOW you need to stop but can't seem to let go of?

ANYTHING BUT FUNCTIONAL

About seven years ago, I was being treated for a "functional" condition irritable bowel syndrome. The only problem was, I couldn't function. I was calling out of work, canceling plans, not showing up for my family. I was a freaking hot mess. I tried one medication and another and another. Nothing worked.

My doctor decided to do a full workup to make sure we weren't missing anything. I was happy and scared at the same time, hoping they would find something that was treatable.

I came out of the anesthesia to hear my doctor say,

"Samantha, everything looks fine. I will see you in my office in a month."

Shut the front door.

I was not waiting four weeks. I went back two weeks later, crying and screaming there was something really wrong with me and it was scaring the crap out of me (literally).

That is when I knew something had to give. I started doing my own research and then educated my doctors about my condition, which was psychological, emotional, and hormonal.

This is the true definition of IBS, my doctor told me.

So why the heck did he wait so long to mention this? He said patients don't respond well when they are told their symptoms start in their heads. I didn't care where it came from. I wanted it GONE so I started on a journey to get my life back, and I didn't stop until I was feeling 99 percent better.

I use that same knowledge to walk my clients down the path to freedom, confident they have the support of someone who has been in their shoes.

Was there ever a time in YOUR life when you struggled with a medical issue and were given the runaround?

YOU'RE FIRED

I have been let go from more jobs than I care to admit.

Why?

I can't seem to play by the rules. I want things MY way. I want to be there when my family needs me. When I decided to stop taking entry-level jobs that stressed me out and kicked up my IBS, it felt crazy scary.

Admitting I couldn't deal with certain situations made me feel like a failure. Then I slowly started to feel better. I did some major soul searching. "What do I want to be when I grow up (again)?

After a week of not working, I registered at the Institute for Integrative Nutrition. I loved every minute of the year-long course. I was going to help people that were suffering like I was. My heart and stomach were happy.

Friends and family thought I was nuts starting a new career at 43.

So, I made some new friends. People that believed in my dreams. They lift me up every day.

I stopped allowing negativity into my life. Huge thanks to my tribe. You know who you are.

What do you need to let go of to live a healthier, happier life?

THE PLAN

I always needed a plan.

10 years ago, I was teaching dance, choreographing and working my sales job on the side.

We were living in our dream house with a 3rd bedroom so our family could grow.

Everything was going exactly as I had planned.

Until it didn't.

We would remain a family of 3.

Working late nights and weekends wasn't the ideal situation raising a 5-year-old.

My dance career came abruptly to an end. My whole plan was unraveling.

I felt like a convict let out after serving 20 years. What the heck do people do all day? How will I remember to brush my teeth?

I started going to the gym every day. Having coffee with friends, driving my son to activities.

Holy crap! This is what it feels like to have a life.

I let go of my plan and enjoyed the journey. It led to many amazing places along the way.

What would I like to tell my 33-year-old self?

Life does not come with a guarantee. Enjoy every minute of every day, and good things will come to you if you let them.

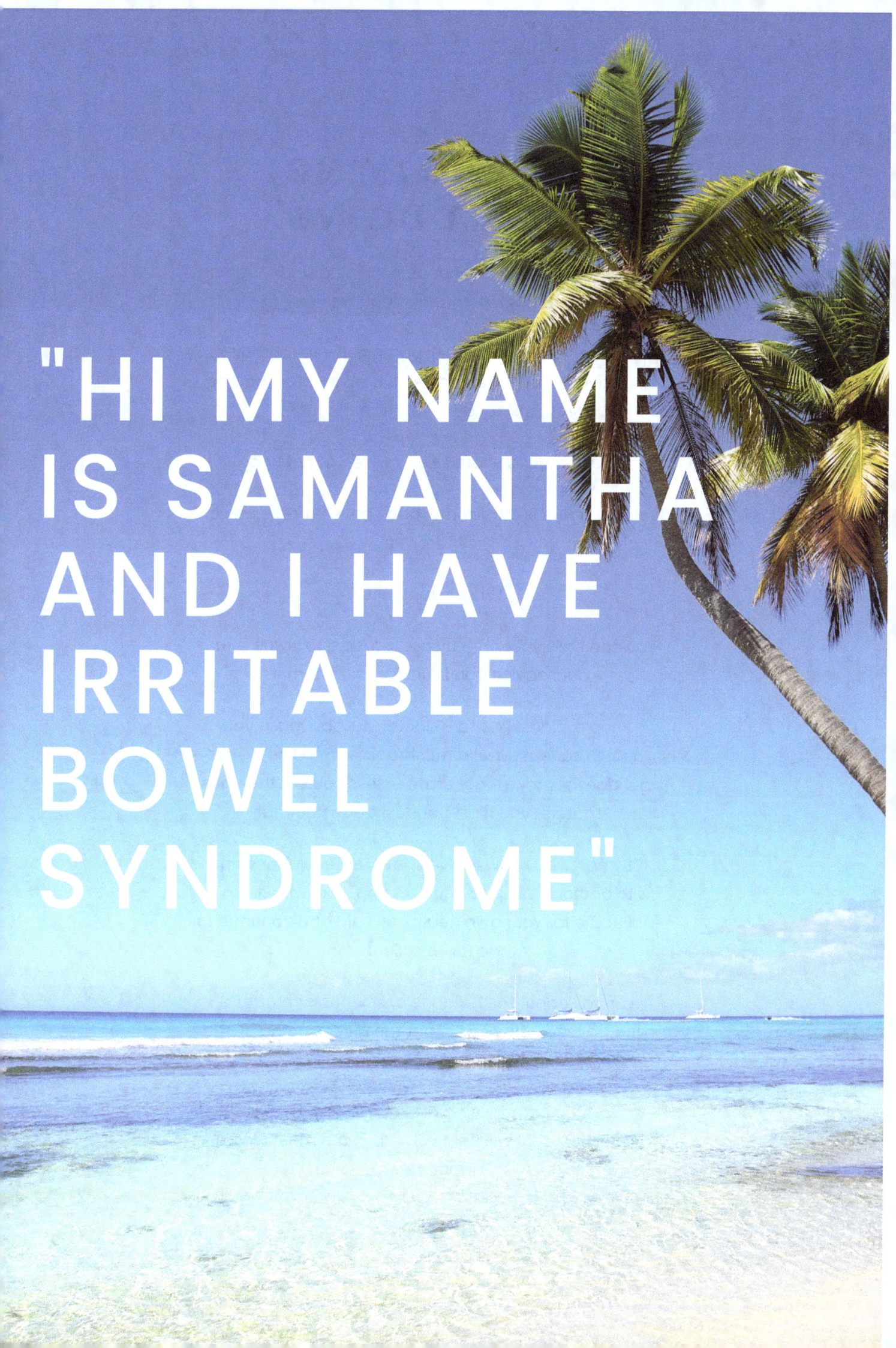

"HI MY NAME IS SAMANTHA AND I HAVE IRRITABLE BOWEL SYNDROME"

STOP TALKING, START DOING

I am so sick and tired of people whining and moaning about their chronic health issues.

I have been in many support groups for chronic digestive disorders, and after five minutes of reading, my anxiety goes through the roof.

These groups should be run like AA meetings:

"Hi, my name is Samantha, and I have irritable bowel syndrome."

(Insert applause)

You can earn your chip by not listening to some numb nuts advice you found on the internet.

People, please, go to a doctor. Just because you heard that eating wild mushrooms would heal your gut doesn't make it accurate unless you eat the ones that get you high. Seriously, don't do that.

By now, you know I have a love/hate relationship with doctors. It's up to you how you work with them to advocate for your own health, as I did and continue to do for my clients.

I am all about the balance of science and nature, and I love to help people put the pieces of the puzzle together.

So, stop complaining and start living. Here is a worksheet that will help you make the most of your appointment.

WHAT I WISH I KNEW
BEFORE VISITING MY DOCTOR

Your personal checklist!

- [ ] Start a daily journal of your symptoms including what you ate, any stress you might be feeling, or any unusual changes.

- [ ] Do research about your specific symptoms, using reliable medical resources like Mayo Clinic or Johns Hopkins.

- [ ] Make a list of questions you want to ask your doctor. Keep a list handy and add to it as things come up. Don't be afraid to be incredibly detailed about how you are feeling and remember nothing is irrelevant. Bring your list to the appointment and make notes. If you are unclear about something, ask again.

- [ ] Medications: ask detailed questions about any prescriptions or over the counter medications including the desired result and any side effects. Research them (reliable sources, see above), before heading to the pharmacy.

- [ ] Do not make too many changes at the same time or you will never know what is working and what's not. Add or subtract things gradually and keep journaling how you feel.

- [ ] Last and most important, you don't need to wait six to eight weeks to follow up with your doctor. If you have a bad reaction, call them right away. If not, give it a week or so and if you are not feeling better, or you feel worse, make another appointment.

BALANCE

Managing functional digestive disorders like IBS is kinda like learning to walk on a balance beam.

You need support, balance and confidence.

In the beginning, you might fall a lot. I sure as heck did. But keep in mind:

*   **Over time, you learn what foods and lifestyle situations knock you down.**

*   **You learn to eat foods that give you strength.**

*   **You know when it's time to use medication and what medication is right for you.**

Eventually, you make it across the beam, head held high without a single wobble.

That victory gives you the confidence to walk that beam again and again. Will you fall sometimes?

Yup.

Just not every time.

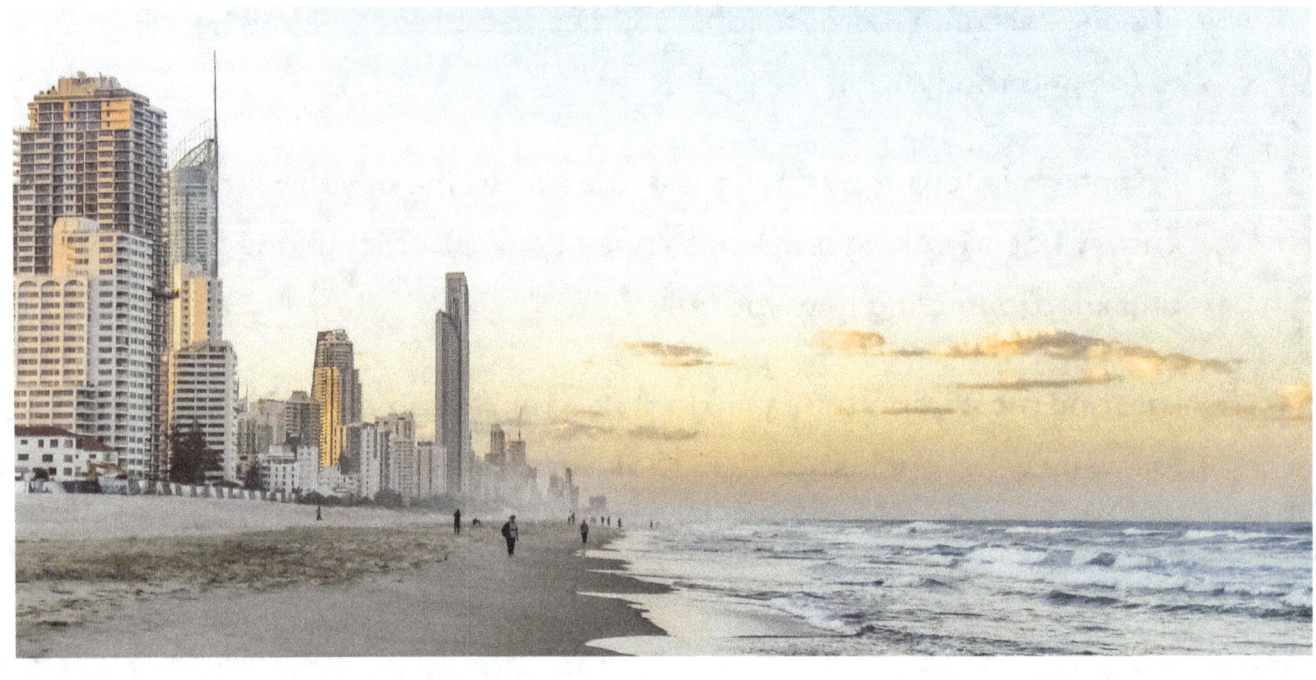

LOUD AND PROUD

Back in my sales days, we had a saying, "the 1st rule about (the company) is no one talks about (the company)'.

My husband likes to call it drinking the Kool-aid.

Three of us suffered from chronic illnesses. We never said a peep (except to each other).

We would get up, dress up, show up every day and do our job as expected.

The medical world expects us to drink their "Kool-aid" or whatever treatment or medication they are selling at the time.

Have you ever felt intimidated by the doctor, like you knew something didn't jibe?

What did you do about it?

Let's break the rules and TALK about it.

FREEDOM

I was never an excellent student in school. Due to various health issues, I was thought to be less than intelligent, so not much was expected of me.

So, like anyone else, I delivered the bare minimum. I set my expectations low since it was drilled into me that I would not be successful. (This was the start of my anxiety and digestive issues.)

Until I was.

I started to question why people assumed I was less than capable.

Something inside me knew I had to work twice as hard as everyone else to get where I want to be, so I dug my heels in.

I found out they were wrong. I was a brilliant child. My communication skills were way above average.

I used this knowledge to break free from the corner I was in. (Do you know that movie?)

At 32, I directed a ballet school and company.

At 38, I was making full-time pay for part-time work in sales.

At 41, I went back to school. Two years later, I started my own business.

If you take away anything from this, know you are not your past. Whatever people thought of you doesn't matter.

All that matters is what you think.

What you want.

You got this!

CH-CH-CH-CHANGES

"What if I try a different approach and I feel worse?"

That is precisely the thing I asked myself, which is why for years I kept the same routine, the exact same food, continuing my search for a "cure."

I was terrified to make any drastic changes; afraid I would no longer be me.

Full disclosure, if you don't make dramatic changes, the suffering will go on and on. The pain, the fear and the shame.

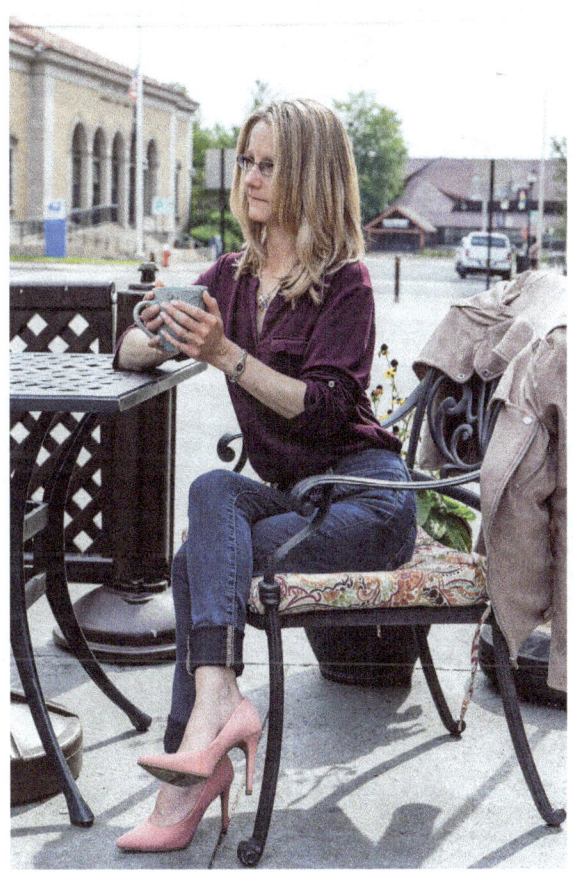

When you decide to unlearn everything you know and seek the root cause of your condition, THAT'S when things start to change for the better.

It doesn't happen overnight. There is an adjustment period. It's almost like being reborn. Once you fight your way out of the darkness (with a little push) a whole new world appears in front of your eyes.

You become the best version of yourself again.

Trust me.

You don't have to feel this way.

OPTIONS

I don't believe in settling. There are multiple solutions to every problem, but you have to be proactive and explore your options.

I made an expensive choice a few years back. It was a Sunday morning. I came downstairs to the coffee pot and before it had brewed, the pain in my abdomen washed over me, and I went down.

I was seen by a Doogie Howser-looking resident in the ER. His first advice was to give me meds to stop the pain (priceless).

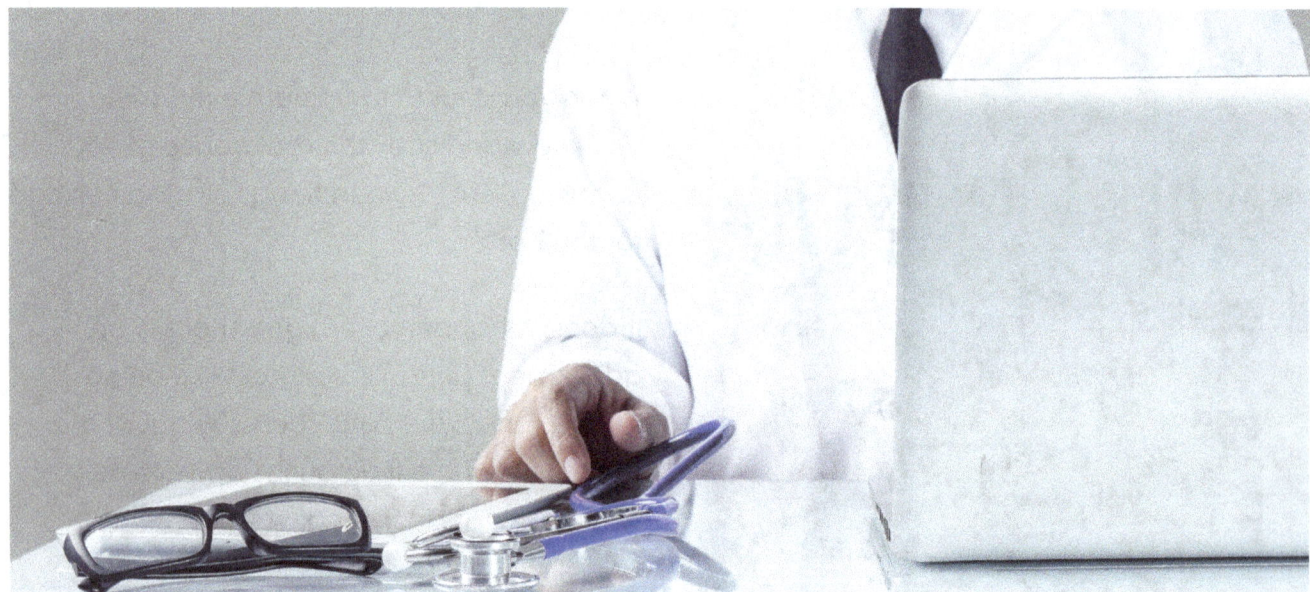

His second was I have a CAT-Scan to rule out appendicitis. I had been back and forth to the doctor and had enough tests to know that was NOT the case.

Yet out of fear, I agreed.

It came back negative (ya think?) with a hefty bill attached.

Looking back now, I would still go to the ER for that level of pain, but I would trust my instincts when it came to the proper course of treatment.

Sorry Doogie.

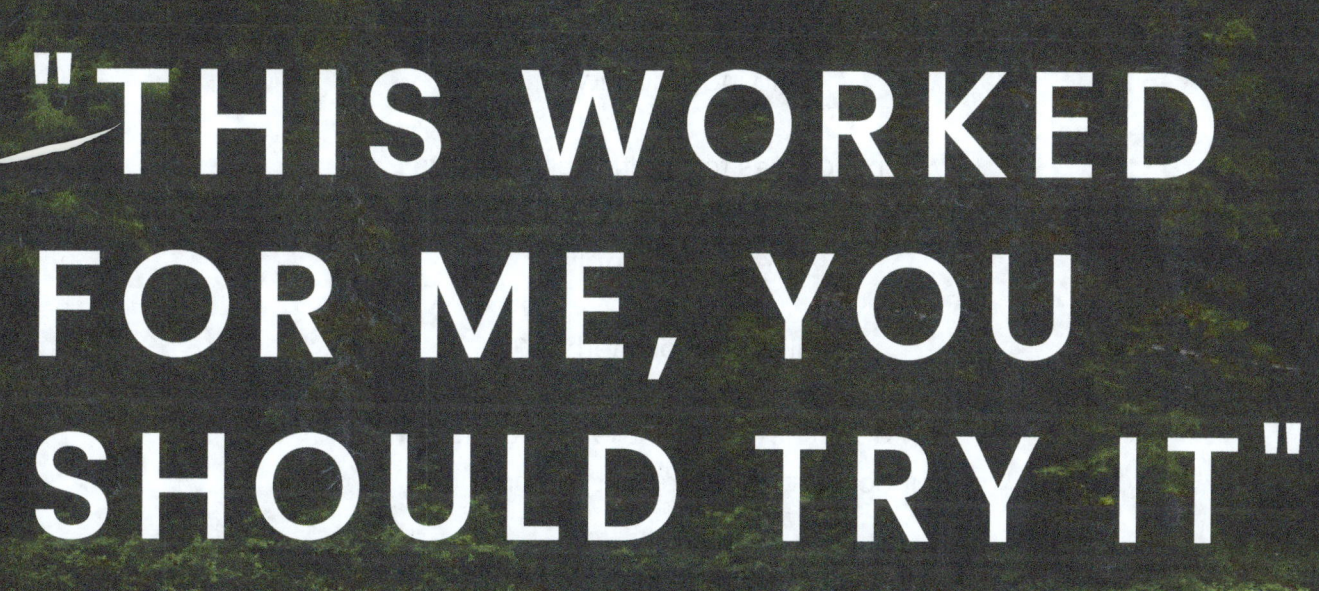

EVERYONE ELSE
IS DOING IT

"This worked for me. You should try it."

"We will just keep trying you on different medications and see how you do."

No. No. No.

Why am I saying no to this approach? Bio individuality.

When it comes to functional digestive disorders, no one thing will work for the same two people.

Trial and error method?

How about "let's get to the root cause of your condition and treat it accordingly?"

It IS possible once you stop believing the hype and get on a better path to freedom.

You DON"T have to feel this way. (If I don't, neither should you.)

I was three steps away from a padded room, you know that feeling?

You can learn to ASK the right questions, TRUST your instincts and TAKE the reins.

Forget about functioning and start living your best life!

IT'S NOT JUST ABOUT FOOD

The reason I chose the Institute for Integrative Nutrition for my certification is their unique approach.

They teach students to explore everything both on and off the plate.

That is so critical when it comes to managing digestive disorders.

I don't write meal plans for my clients, although I will send them recipes upon request.

When I work with clients, I listen and ask them high-mileage questions like, "tell me more about that" or "how did that make you feel?"

When I stopped obsessing about food being the trigger for my digestive issues, I realized there was WAY more involved.

I would be happy to tell you more.

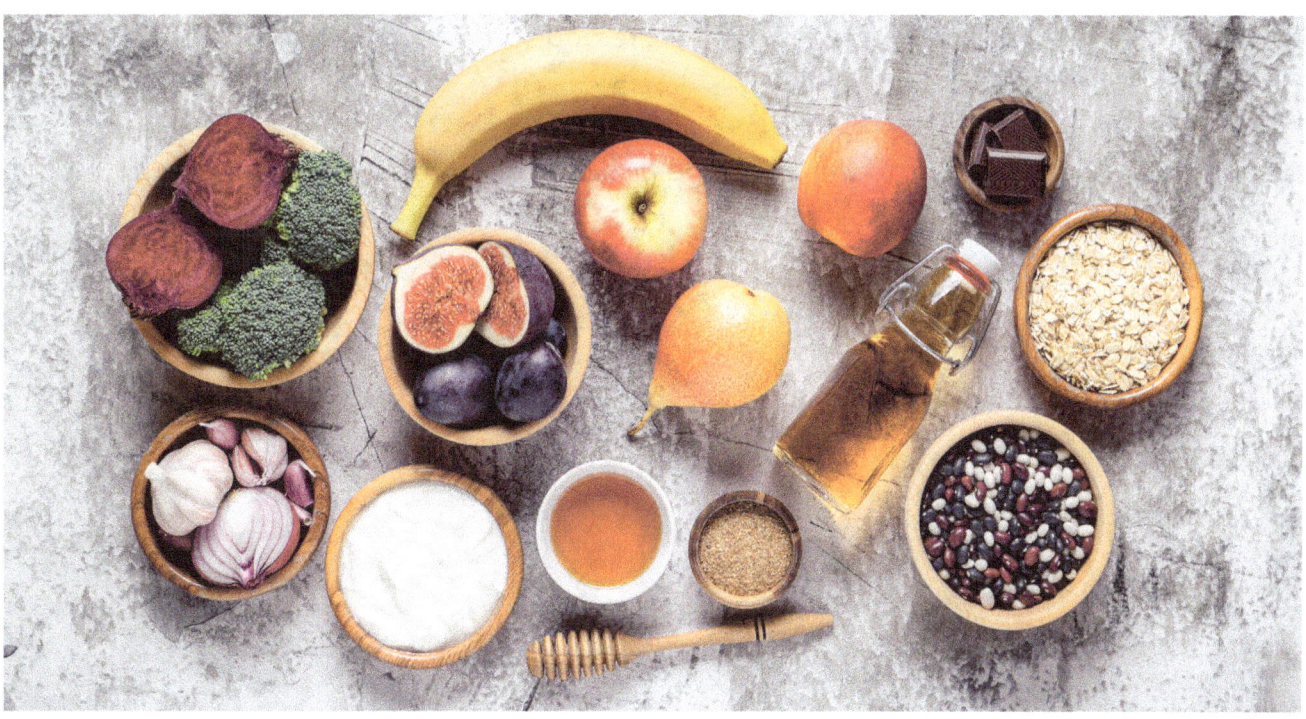

LIVE YOUR BEST LIFE

Many choices I made to treat the root cause of my chronic digestive disorder raised a few eyebrows in my circle.

Many of my friends were experiencing similar issues, yet they chose to continue suffering.

We only have one life to live. You can bet your derriere I want to feel my best.

Not better.

Not good enough.

My BEST life.

My friend Tom Martin calls it the "fast burn" and the "slow burn." (credit Patty Lennon)

I am not a patient woman. Once I found the root cause of my condition, I went for the "fast burn" and watched my symptoms reduce in just a few months.

The "slow burn" involved having the energy to change my diet and lifestyle.

Now thanks to the balance of science and nature and some scary steps into the unknown, I am the best version of myself that I have EVER been.

It's not the "WHAT" that will improve your digestive disorders. It's the WHY.

What's your WHY?

CHOICES

Knowledge is power.

The more you educate yourself about your health issues, the more choices you have.

I am a HUGE believer in choices. Anyone that knows me knows I never see anything as black or white.

I like to live dangerously, in the gray area (except when it comes to my hair, lol).

Yes, I want to live a life free from digestive issues, but I want to ENJOY my life.

When you know all the options, you can decide what works best for your life. No one thing works for the same two people.

What choices have YOU made that allow you to live your best life?

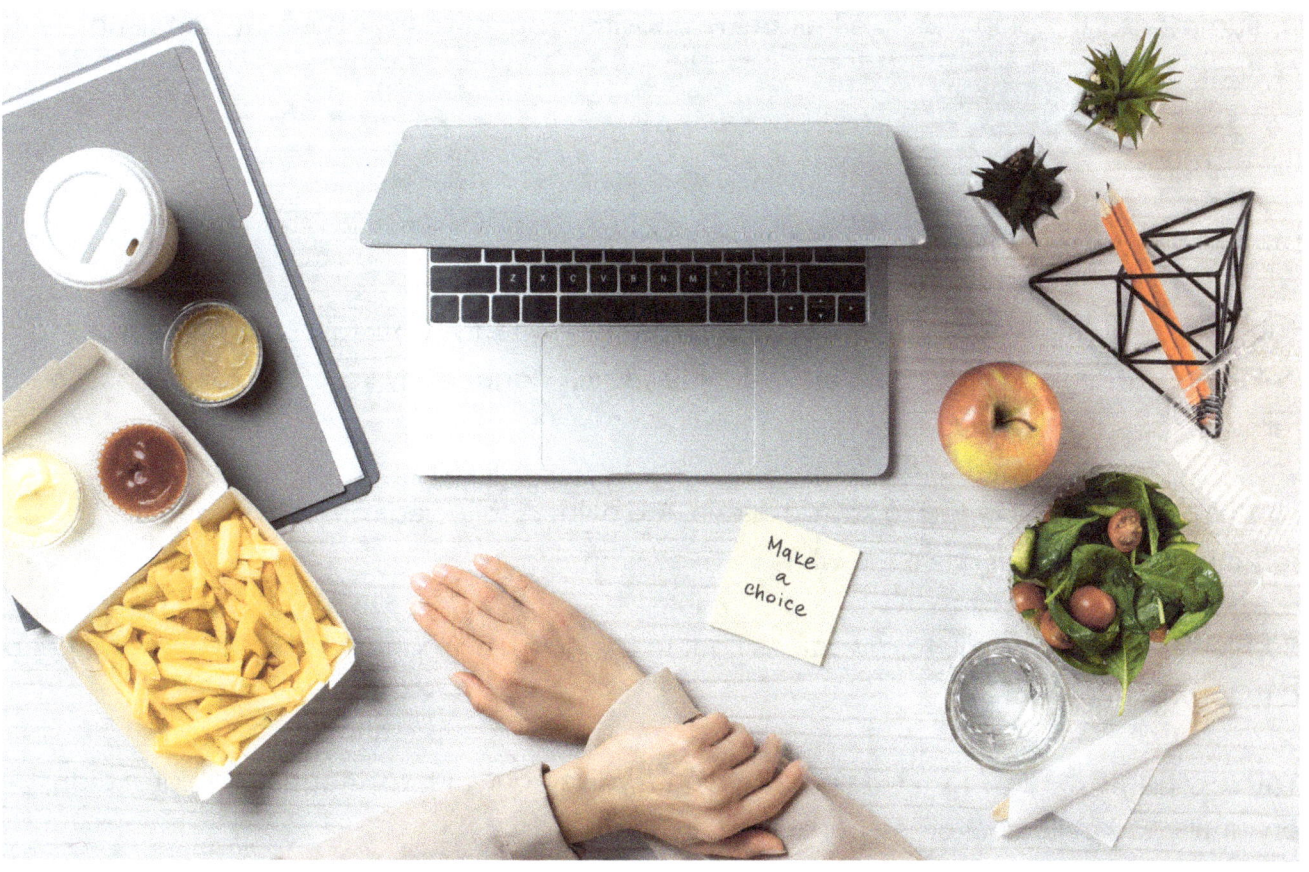

LIFE HAPPENS

I was on my way to work when I got the text.

"Both owners are here in a closed room with the office manager."

She was already gone by the time I got there.

I was the client recruiter, the one who worked tediously to schedule portraits, and I had a killer track record. Without clients, there would be no sales, without sales, no money, so I had to be safe, right?

I went to my desk and unpacked my things, shaking as I logged into the system and pretended to read emails.

"Samantha, can we talk to you for a minute?"

I prayed they would tell me about the office manager being let go and what the new plan was.

To summarize, the plan was to eliminate my position, but it wasn't about my performance or dedication.

It was money.

I stared them straight in the eyes and said NOTHING.

They watched me like a criminal as I turned over all my leads and collected my personal belongings that I had accumulated over nine years. I handed my keychain to my boss to remove my office key since I shook too much.

I had one request. I wanted to say goodbye. The owners followed me as I hugged the remaining staff. My friends cried while I stayed stone-faced.

Both owners escorted me to my car. As I got to the door, my manager said, "if you ever need a recommendation..."

With my hand on the door, I said goodbye and walked out with my head held high. I didn't cry until I had pulled out of the parking lot.

What did it mean for me? FREEDOM. No more manipulating clients with smoke and mirrors. No more telling lies. I had gotten so good at my pitch, it was making me sick.

I was eligible for unemployment since I got fired, which allowed me to explore what I wanted to do next. I wanted to help people. REALLY help them. Not just organize a 45-minute family gathering that had the potential to cost them thousands.

That is how I got here. A certified Integrative Nutrition Health Coach dedicated to helping people with functional digestive disorders get back to work, back to enjoying food, traveling, and enjoying quality time with family and friends.

What impact is your job having on your health?

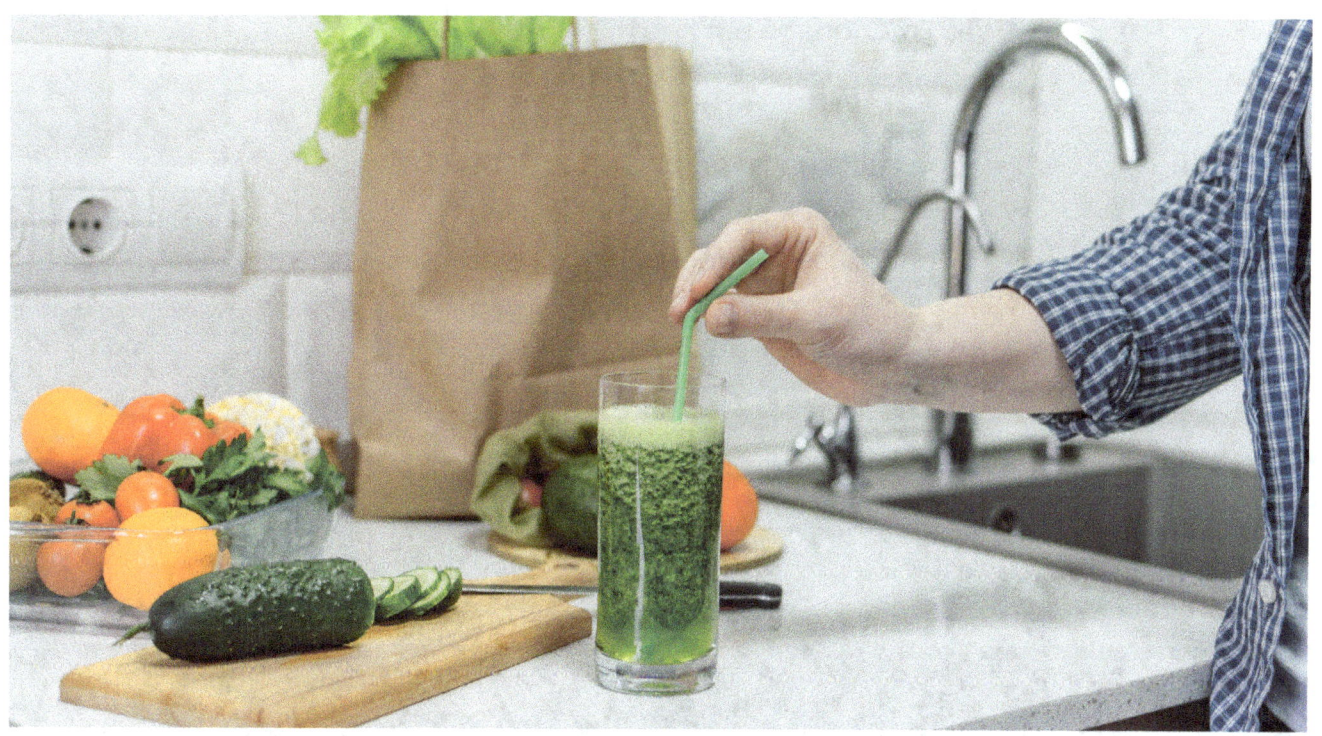

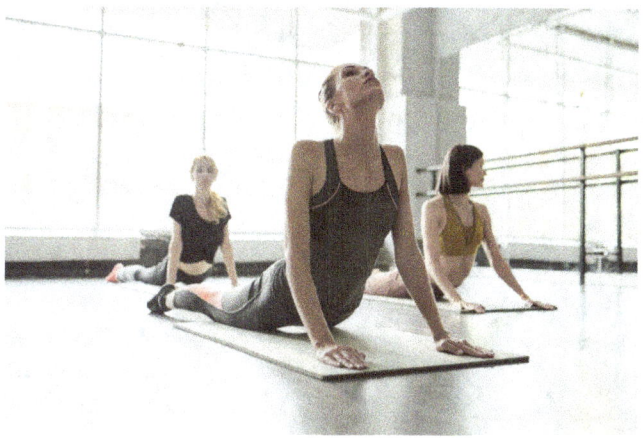

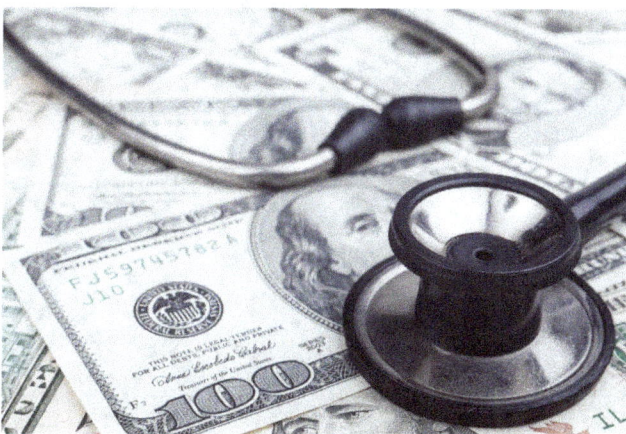

NO ONE IS PERFECT

I don't really enjoy cooking.

I am a terrible driver.

I get Botox.

I like (no, love) wine.

I have 2 tattoos.

Yet, I manage to eat healthily and stay healthy despite my imperfections.

You don't need to sit around all day meditating and baking kale chips to function with IBS. Once you find the root cause and identify triggers, there will be wiggle room for some fun things, like cake and wine.

What's your guilty pleasure?

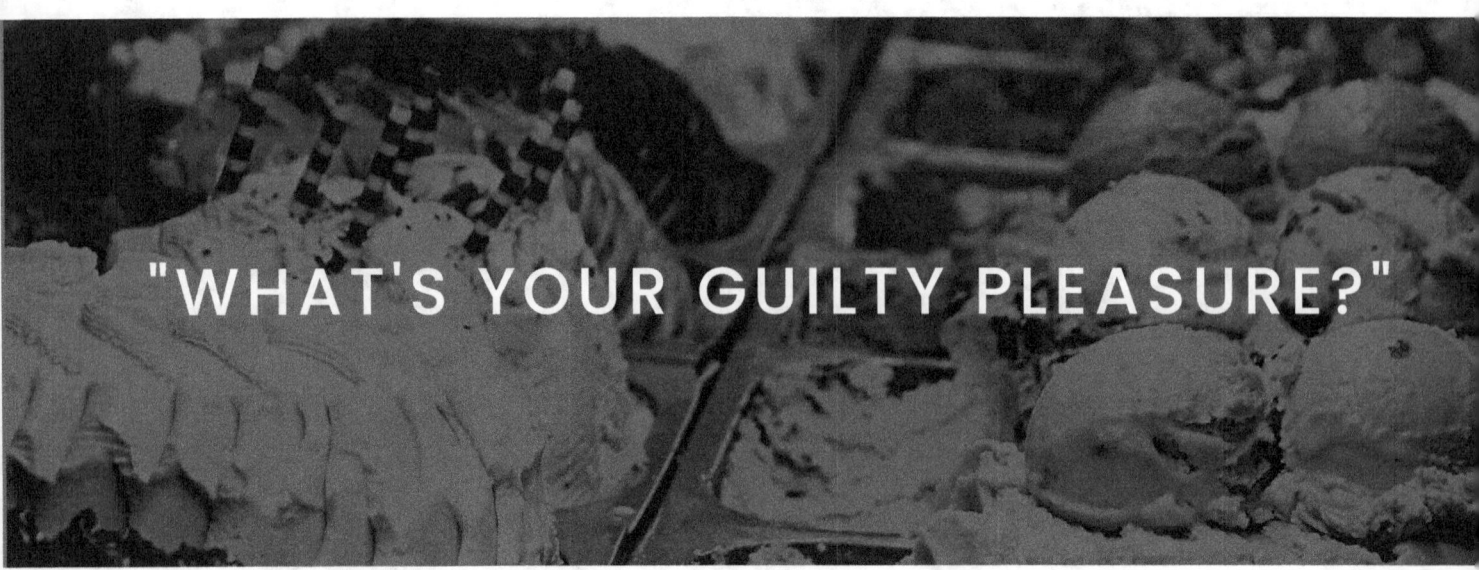

"WHAT'S YOUR GUILTY PLEASURE?"

THE WHY

Managing functional digestive disorders is like peeling away the layers of an onion.

There is no "quick fix" or "magic pill".

Your doctor does not have enough time to spend with you to ask about your diet, lifestyle, career or family life.

ALL THE THINGS that lead to chronic digestive disorders. It is easier for them to keep prescribing different medications and collecting your money.

What can you do? Eliminate the top 5 triggers for two weeks: gluten, sugar, dairy, eggs, and soy.

After 14 days, start reintroducing these things, one at a time, into your diet and see how you feel.

Not everyone has the same triggers, so you may be surprised what makes you feel fine and what makes you feel like crap.

I ate nothing but bananas and rice crackers for months before I discovered the root cause of my condition.

If you eliminate all of these things and don't feel the slightest bit better, it's time to look at managing your stress, improving your relationships and bringing more joy into your life.

Not sure where to start?

I got you.

THE HOW

How do we find relief from digestive disorders without the runaround?

You might have doctors who are trying different medications without looking for the root cause, leaving you tired of the side effects, and the constant back and forth.

This is where becoming your own health advocate can help. How do we do this?

1. **Keep a journal of what you eat, how you feel, and anything unusual that happened. (Stress at work, fight with your spouse)**

2. **Do your research. Again, you'll want to use reputable sources like the Mayo Clinic or Johns Hopkins for information and natural remedies for your symptoms.**

3. **Bring all this information to your doctor. If your doctor is not receptive to these ideas, look for a functional medicine doctor that can get you on the path to recovery.**

After YEARS of trial and error, back and forth, I did my own research and then educated my doctors about the root cause of my condition.

Once we treated the root cause, it was all downhill from there!

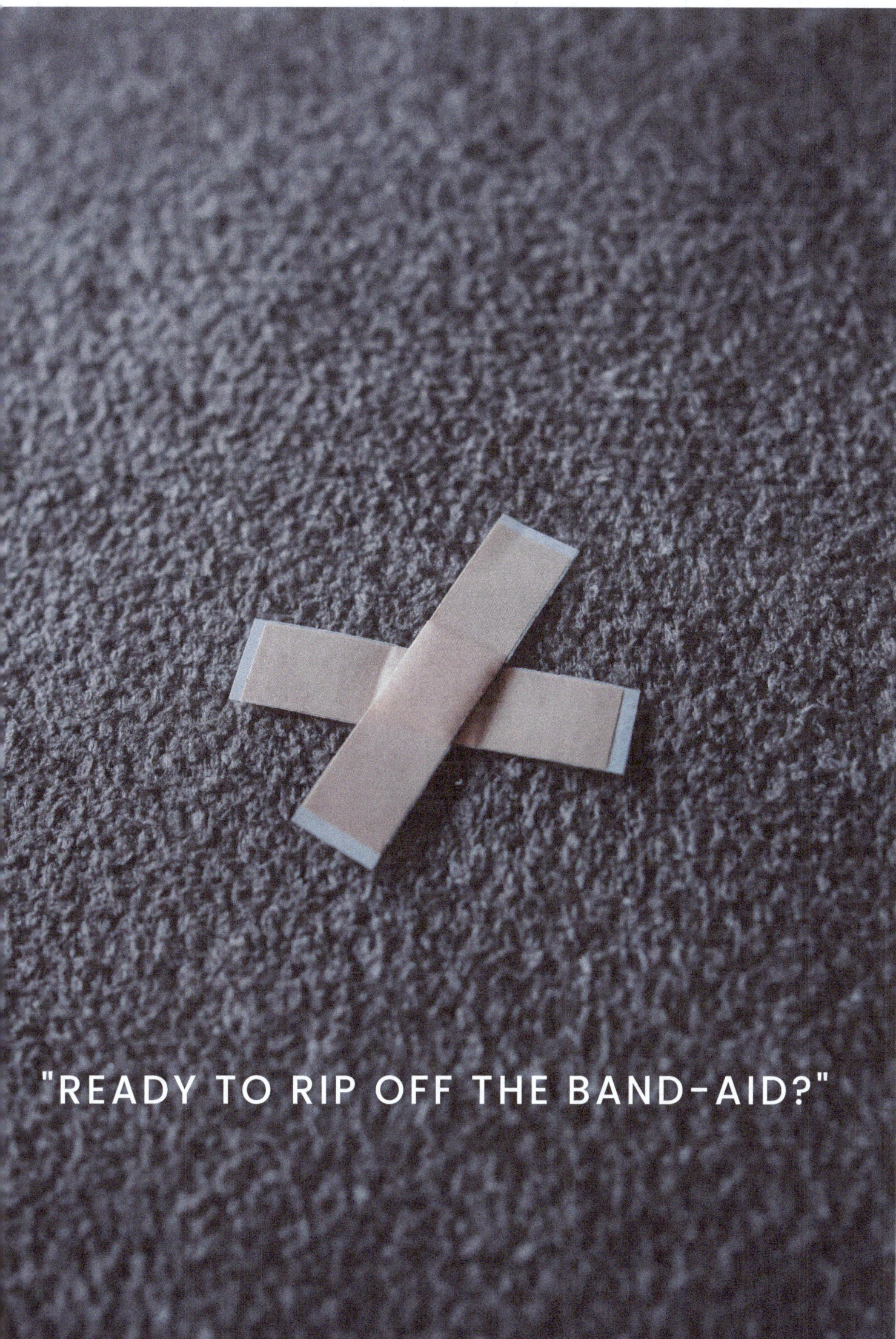

"READY TO RIP OFF THE BAND-AID?"

THE BAND-AID APPROACH

I hear this all the time.

"My doctors will figure it out eventually".

If you have a functional digestive disorder, that statement is far from accurate.

If you are searching for freedom from your symptoms, there are many moving parts to consider.

Medication may be the first step in the right direction, but not the ultimate cure.

What else is involved?

Diet, lifestyle, stress, relationships, exercise, to name a few.

Medication is only a Band-Aid. The good news?

Once you do the work to find the root cause or triggers of your condition, a full recovery is totally possible.

Ready to rip off the Band-aid?

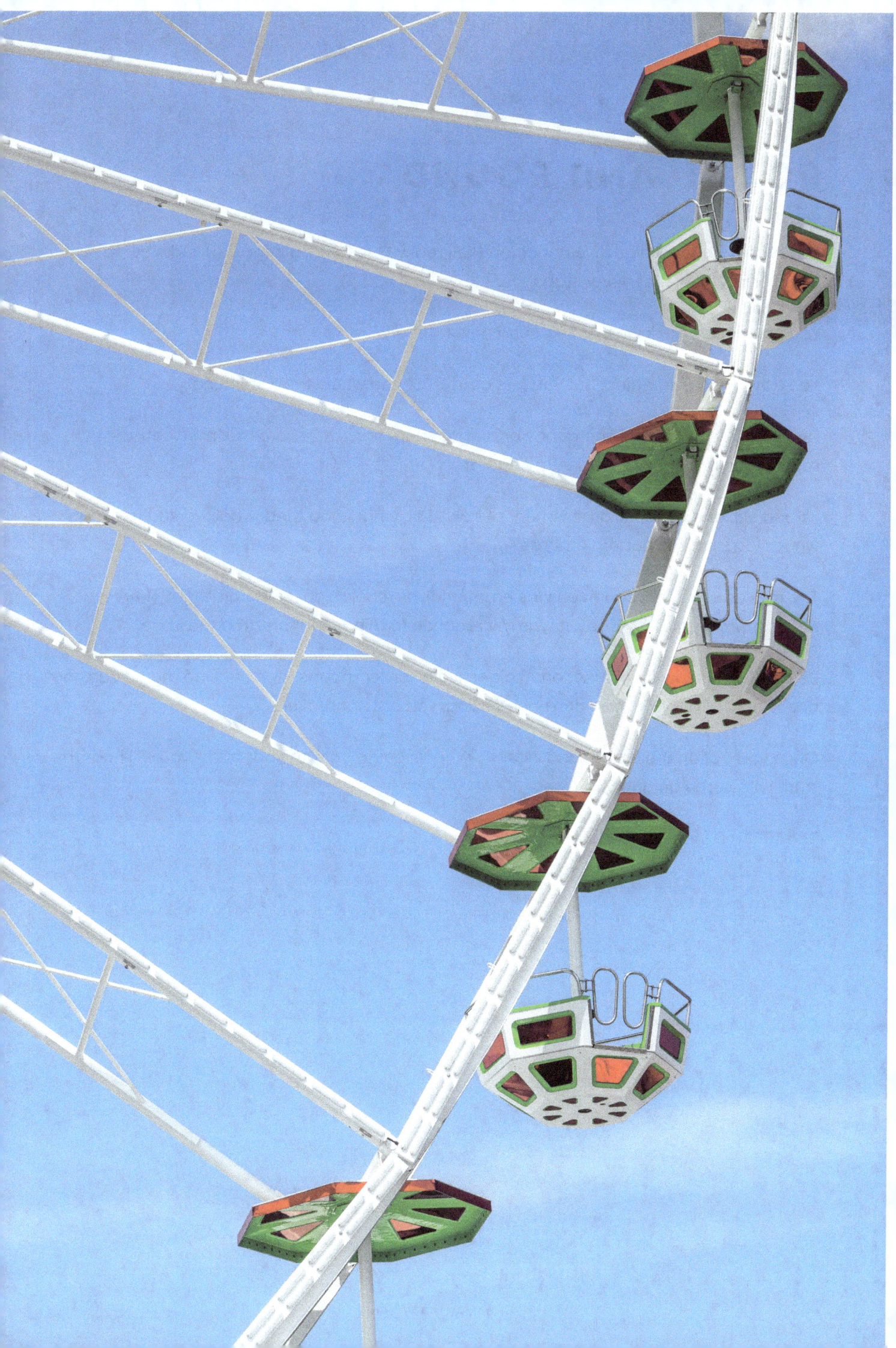

ROUND AND ROUND

Having a functional digestive condition (IBS, Leaky Gut, GERD, ulcers, etc) is like being stuck on a Ferris Wheel that never stops.

You have ups and downs, but you can never get off.

You have tried everything, but you just can't STOP the wheel from spinning.

Five years ago, I hit the emergency brake. NO more tests, NO more trial medications. NO more waiting six months to see my doctor.

I stood still and did a full assessment of how I felt, what I had tried, what worked for what, what didn't. I saw a pattern emerge.

The root cause of my condition was emotional, psychological, and hormonal. There was nothing wrong with my body. It was my reaction to things that created the issue.

Being diagnosed with a "functional" digestive disorder means there was no magic cure, no one magic pill to "fix" it. You don't need fixing. You are not broken.

Once you put on the brakes and listen to what is going on with your body, you will hear the truth with some guidance.

The TRUTH is what sets you free.

"WHAT BOLD STEPS WILL YOU TAKE TO GET YOUR LIFE BACK?"

THERE IS HOPE

Do you dream of a life without your fear and shame from your chronic digestive disorder?

Would you like to wake up and take on the day without wondering whether you would have a flair up?

Do you long to enjoy time with family and friends without being stuck in the bathroom?

Believe me, I have been there and done that, and I promise YOU CAN!

Be an advocate for your health, keep a diary of your symptoms, ask someone to help you connect the dots. Challenge your doctors. You don't have to live this way!

Functional digestive disorders are not a life sentence. You CAN get control and live the life you have been dreaming of.

What bold steps will you take to get your life back?

NOURISH YOURSELF

These days, I eat things my stomach could never handle, like fruit.

Who knew it was so good?

Also, I love me a good salad packed with superfoods like kale, beets and pumpkin seeds, things I never could have digested five years ago

What foods do I shy away from now? Processed foods, sugar, too much gluten.

Do I get the eye roll from my family? Almost every day.

IDC! They do what they do, and I do my own thing.

Bring on the eye rolls. Five years ago, I couldn't hold down water and now I eat healthy, nutritious foods every day.

It may seem impossible for you now, but I PROMISE if I can get to where I am now, so can you.

THE HARD TRUTH

What does it really mean to overcome a functional digestive disorder?

- **Making choices. Changing something significant in your life so you can enjoy each day.**

- **Staying committed to diet and lifestyle choices that have gotten you to where you are.**

- **Knowing the inevitable if you "fall off the wagon". (I unknowingly ran out of probiotics. I immediately placed an order, thinking "I am doing so well, a few days won't matter." Today I ran to a friend's house to get enough until my order arrived).**

- **Doctors will disagree with you. Big deal. It's your body and your money. Keep fighting.**

- **It's not just about your stomach. You will need to do a deep dive into ALL aspects of your life to get to the root cause. Some of it might not be pretty, but there is light at the end of the tunnel.**

You CAN live a worry-free, pain-free life. You can advance your career, eat foods you love, travel, and enjoy quality time with family and friends.

What's it worth to you?

ABOUT SAMANTHA WYLAND

Samantha is a multiple trauma survivor who suffered physical and emotional issues starting at a very young age. Over the course of 30 years, she has undergone more than 20 operations, including open-heart surgery at the age of nine. Her chronic digestive issues began when she was 16 and was diagnosed with Peptic Ulcers, a Hiatal Hernia, Gastrointestinal Reflux Disease, and Irritable Bowel Syndrome (IBS).

In 1995, Samantha was in a near-fatal accident with many injuries, including multiple skull fractures and a temporal fracture of the inner ear that caused hearing loss and temporary facial paralysis. Her strong desire to graduate college led her to undergo multiple operations to reconstruct her inner ear and numerous plastic surgeries to restore facial symmetry.

Today, Samantha uses the knowledge about health and wellness that she mastered to transform her own life, and the resilience she has developed through this lengthy process, to help others living with chronic digestive disorders. She uses that knowledge to walk her clients down the same path to freedom and an enhanced quality of life, confident they have the support of someone who has been in their shoes.

The information that Samantha shares with others struggling with chronic digestive disorders are the result of a passionate inquiry into solutions to a variety of medical challenges she has encountered in her own life.

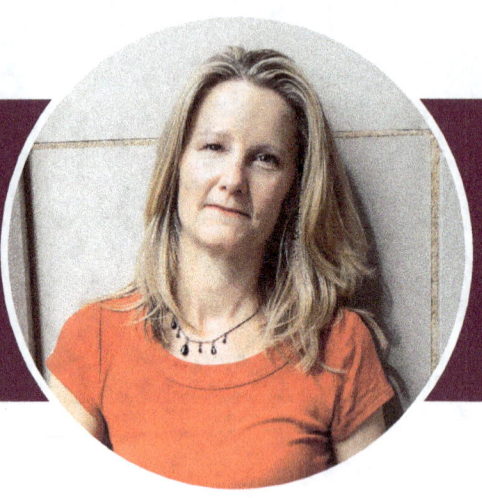

After attending Immaculata High School in 1991 and graduating from DeSales University 1999 with a B.A. in Dance, Samantha began a 20-year career performing, teaching and choreographing ballets with Montgomery Dance that was later renamed The Dance Connection. Samantha performed in and choreographed original ballets locally for children including The Nutcracker, Cinderella, Sleeping Beauty and Beauty and the Beast.

During this time, she got married, surrounded by her students, friends and family. In 2006 she performed in her last ballet, The Nutcracker, 12 weeks pregnant with her son. She retired in 2012 to focus on her family and raise her son, then five.

From 2006-2015 she worked in sales at Kramer Portraits. In 2019 she Studied Integrative Nutrition and health coaching at Institute for Integrative Nutrition. Samantha and her husband live in New Jersey with their son and their miniature poodle, Leo.

To learn more about Samantha Wyland and her health coaching services, visit:

www.yourbestlifebysamantha.com

Your Best Life *by Samantha*

DESIGNED BY WWW.HINDMARSHPRODUCTIONS.COM

www.ingramcontent.com/pod-product-compliance
Lightning Source LLC
Chambersburg PA
CBHW081202280526
45791CB00007B/2168

* 9 7 8 1 3 8 7 5 3 9 0 7 9 *